Birds in the sky

Birds in the sky fly high above.
Soaring high.
Feeling a freedom many of us want to feel.
Why can't we feel that freedom today?
Sure we can't fly, but we don't need to fly
to feel a freedom so fine.
Freedom is not only high above, it's right here too.
It's able to talk, able to laugh, able to do things you enjoy.
So in many ways we are those birds, in the sky, who feel that freedom.
But most of all, freedom is in all of us.

I close my eyes

I close my eyes.
I just don't want to see.
I close my eyes.
I need to take a moment.
I close my eyes.
I breathe deeply.
I feel every vibe. I connect.
I close my eyes to have a moment
to feel a space that helps me move on.
Whenever I need to take a moment I close my eyes.

I close my eyes.

I'm here for you

I'm here for you.
I know I don't always show it.
I'm always here.
Whenever and wherever you need me.
I'm here for you.

When you want to talk or just a hug.
I'm there for you.
You have given me so much and keep on giving.
Not just now, but always.
I'm here for you.

My road is long

My road is long.
I am not even half way down.
I look back down the road.
I can see what I've been through.

I see all the lessons I've learnt.
I see happiness and sadness.
I see achievements, struggles and pain.

I look forward to the long road ahead.
I can't see what is waiting for me at every corner.
All I can see is a long road full of twists and turns.

The road may be long but I have my head up high,
With the knowledge of what's behind me
I can use it on the long road ahead.

My road is long.

Don't you know?

Don't you know we are always there for you?
We are always there when you call us.

Don't you know we see your good and bad times?
We always leave a sign that we been there with you.

Don't you know how much we help you make the right choices?
Just listen and connect with us because we want you to know.

Don't you know?

You are just you

You are just you.
The shy person, always trying to please.

You are just you.
Nobody is the same as you.
You are not a disappointment.
Don't be afraid.

You are just you.
Say what you feel.
Do what you think is right for you.
Don't care about what others think.

You are just you.
You have your life to live.
Your life is your own.
Do what is best for you.

Everyone follows a path,
We learn lessons.
But you are just you.
So don't care what others think about you.
It is only their way of thinking
They are not you.

You are just you
Unique.
You are who you are.
You are just you.

They

They walk behind me to push me along.

They walk next to me to support me.

They walk in front of me to guide me.

They are always there wanting the best for me.

They won't judge me when I make mistakes.

They are my spirit guides. They are my helpers. They are my family.

They are with you too.
They guide you. They help you.

They tell you what's good and bad.

They won't judge you.

They are just there when you are ready to listen.

They

Just the way we are

Just the way we are.
What is wrong with the way we are?
Nothing is wrong.

Still we want to change things.
When we are not happy about something.
We want to change it.

Some want to be slim.
Some want a six-pack.
You name it!
How about simply accepting,
just the way we are ?

We are all born special.
You know that makes you perfect.
We are all influenced by our family, and our friends.
It will play on your mind and you will try to change it.
Just the way we are.

There is nothing wrong with change or changing yourself.
It may be a contradiction.
Just the way we are.

I bring you this simple message.
We are who we are.
We are all special in our own way.
People will just have to accept us
just the way we are.

Light and darkness

There was darkness for a long time.

Then there was light.

The light stayed for years but then started to go.

Darkness returned and battled with the light.

Sometimes darkness won.

Sometimes the light won.

Now they are both here and life is in perfect harmony.

There is no light without darkness and there is no darkness without light.

There is just the perfect balance.

Could you send me an angel?

Could you send me an angel?
Not for me but for everyone who needs one.
For everyone who needs help.
For everyone who needs strength to face a new day.

Could you send an angel?
To my friends and family.

Could you send an angel?
To people in poor countries who live without hope.
Let them know they are not alone.

Could you send your angels of sunshine?

So they can feel the warmth.

Could you send your angels of love?

So they can feel the comfort.

Could you send me an angel?

Every day

Every day I am reminded.
Every day is another battle.
Every day I look for hope.
Every day I fight with myself.
Every day I wonder if I'm good enough.
Every day I learn.
Every day I wonder if I love myself.

Every day I fight these thoughts.

But every day they make me stronger.

We always need love.

We don't always get what we want.
Others don't always understand our needs.
In times of need, we all need help.
It does not always mean we need money.
Do we take time to really listen?
Do we fully understand what is said?

Sometimes it's about money but that's not always the problem.
There are so many other things people ask for.
But why do we fear when they ask for help?
Sometimes there are other things people ask for.
Sometimes they just need is a hug and to hear *"I'm here for you"*.
That may be the most important thing you do for someone.
Please listen and pay attention when someone asks for help.

We always need love.

Finding yourself

My questions are simple,
Have you found yourself?
Do you know who you are?
Do you know what your lessons are?

We are here for a purpose.
We were born with a purpose.
To learn.

I have been on this quest and still am.
But I have learned so much.
One of my lessons is to know we are here to understand love.
This is the biggest lesson that we all have to learn.
We are here to learn love because, at the end of the day, your life love still remains.
Yes, we complain, we struggle and we fight.
We are unhappy.
Believe me, I am still struggling with it.
But deep in my heart love is all I need.
So here it goes. Yes, I will have my days but deep inside I love you and I know that's all we need.

Being yourself

Being yourself is so important.
We lose ourselves too much.
We even try to change ourselves.
Why? For what reason?
What's wrong with being the person you are?
Why change?

If you're doing it for yourself, ok, fine, go for it.
Does that not mean that you're happy with yourself?
I understand we go through changes. That's ok.
We are perfect in every way and don't have to change for anyone.

Be complete

You need to know what happiness is and express it.
You need to know what sadness is and express it.
You need to know what hurt is and feel it.
You need to know what love is and experience it.
All this will make you one with yourself and be complete.

I am standing at the window

I'm standing at the window, looking outside.
My mind is going nowhere.
Just staring at a world that keeps going.

While staring, I notice I am standing still,
taking everything in.
I'm just standing there realizing how absorbed we are
in our daily lives.
Things we have to do; work and taking care of others.
Looking out the window I realize these things are normal.
They take up time.
But, we forget to think about ourselves.
We need time for ourselves.
We need time to take care of ourselves.
We need to take time for us as well.

I am standing at the window.
I let everything slow down while the rest is speeding up.
I stand still and take time for myself. Do you?

I am standing at the window.

Trying

Everyday we try to do our best.
To be the best we can. I guess.
We learn by trying and by believing in trying.
It's good to try things even if you fail.
By trying you will learn.
But if you try things with bad intentions you will fail.
You see, trying to make someone believe something that is not true
will come back to haunt you.
So I would like to say try things for the good, not for the bad.
But most of all believe in yourself.
That is the best thing to try.

Trying

Purpose

Everyone has a purpose in life.
The main one is to love yourself and others.

My purpose is spreading calmness and joy.
Calmness to give them peace and joy to make them laugh.

I found my purpose in life. Have you?

Purpose

What they expect

People often expect so much from you.
Sometimes they expect nothing.
What are their expectations?
Not from life but from people?

Why can't our expectations be the same?
Yes, some people will give more than others, but expect little back.
High expectations could put pressure on the person.
Given more or giving less should not be an issue.
It does not make us better or worse than others.
Expect and respect what we can and cannot do.
That is expecting and respecting each other.

What they expect

These hands
These hands have done so much.
Looking at these hands,
I've been taken back to my memories.

These hands have done so much.
They have shaken other hands in good and bad times.
These hands have hugged people who needed it.
These hands have greeted good friends.

These hands do so much.
They go through so much and yet I don't dwell on it.
These hands of mine heal physically and mentally.
They give love.
Just remember, the body part that you use most are your hands.
Not only mine but everybody's hands heal in some way or another.

These hands

I am

I am who I am - That's a famous saying.
What you see is what you get. And I am me.
I am proud to be that person who makes mistakes.
Who tells jokes, who is loving and doesn't think badly of others.
I am that person that gives 100%.
I am that person who cares for you even if you don't care about me.
I may not be the smartest person in the world but, hey, I don't have to be.
Yes, I get hurt by people. I have my moments.
But you know what - *I am who I am.*
I'm special and that's more important then anything else.

I am

Candle

A candle was given to us the day we are born.
We might not see this candle but it's there.
Burning brightly.
Like every other candle, the wax melts and the candle gets shorter and shorter.
We know this but don't think about it.

Every candle is special so that makes you special.
It does not matter who you are, what you are or what you have. You are still that candle.
A candle is like everybody else.
It does not matter if you are rich or poor.
It does not matter if you are famous or not.
It does not matter if you are sick or not.
It is important to enjoy life and learn.

We all go through many things no matter your status.
Everyone is equal.
So whatever state you're in try to make the best of it.
Be happy. Enjoy life.

Don't let your candle burn out without knowing you are loved.
Knowing that we are all the same.
Knowing that we are here to help.
Most of all let yourself feel loved everyday.
Don't let your candle go out without a fight.
Candle

Can you take me back?

Can you take me back?
I always think about you.
I know you are always there for me.
Even though I don't see you, I know you are there.

I know I should not have done what I did, but you are always there.
You're so close and yet so far away.
I know it's up to me.
I know I did not surrender.
Now I don't see you any more and yet I feel you.
Always reminding me that you're still there.
Letting me know where my destiny lies.
Letting me know what I should be doing.

Give me some time to appreciate how much I had.
Walking behind and always following.
I will come back if you still want me.
Let me recognize you again.
Let me feel you again and I will do what I need to do.

Can you take me back?

I'm just a boat

I'm just a boat starting my journey.
From the harbour I call my mother.
I set out to the ocean that is my path of life.
The ocean takes the boat in every direction.

I face calmness, and storms that take me off course.
This course will lead me to a better understanding.
Sometimes I let myself be carried but other times I will resist.

The ocean will have always storms for me
but there will be sunshine too.
I will survive whatever comes my way.
I always make it back to the harbour.

I'm just a boat

The Maze

Life is like a maze.
We begin our journey at birth.
During our time in the maze
we lose our way in sadness and despair
through which many lessons are learned.

As we grow, we get wiser and enjoy our time
having fun and being happy.
Finally when we reach the end of the maze
we feel complete and a mission accomplished.

As we exit the maze we realize that although we have had bad and sad moments
It was by not giving up that we found a way out.

Clouds

There are clouds in the sky.
These clouds come in every shape and form.
Clouds can predict so many things.
But when look up at the clouds
we only think that it might rain.
Why don't we look at the shape or form?
When we look closer we can see things in them.
It's a fantasy.
A whole different world.
A fantastic world that is accessible to us, if we use our imagination.
Clouds can be so more then just a weather prediction.

Clouds

Slowly

Slowly.
I know it's happening.
Slowly.
I see it coming.
Slowly.
It's creeping closer.
Slowly.
I am the only one who sees it.
Slowly.
I prepare myself. It's coming.
Slowly.
The signs are showing and slowly I give in.
Slowly.
Wondering if I'll ever be ready.
Slowly.
I know I am but slowly I wonder.

Slowly

Stranger

You knew me once before.
Now you lost me.
Busy in a world that does not belong to you.
A world where I do not exist.

Find me.
I'll meet you half way.
You are my path now and forever.
We became strangers because I did not understand.
Did not want to learn.
I was stupid.
Strange things have happened and stranger things will cross our path.
You are my perfect stranger.
I can deal with being strange as we're all strangers.
Keep on fighting stranger because one day you will not be a stranger anymore.

Stranger

Just a hug

A hug can do so many things.
Just a hug can let you know that everything is going to be all right.
Letting you know that you are there and caring for each other.
Just a hug to let you know you're not alone.

The power of a hug is so intense.
It's saying more then words ever can describe.
Just a hug.
Just to feel its power.

We all need a hug not only when we're sad or going through a rough time.
But, also when we love someone.
You know somebody needs it.
For some people it's just a hug but for others it means so much more.
We all need a hug sometimes.

Just a hug

Life is our puzzle.

Life is like a puzzle.
Every little piece of the puzzle
represents every step of our life.

Sometimes we get stuck
not knowing where the pieces fit
in the puzzle.

We stop for a while but then continue on.
It's hard not to give up and get the puzzle done.

Life is a puzzle.
We don't know all the answers but,
when we keep on trying the pieces will fall into place.

Our life is a puzzle.
We keep on trying till our puzzle is complete.

Life is our puzzle.

You're not me

You're not me.
I don't want you to be.
You are who you are.
Good. Bad.

You're not me.
But I'm the same like you.
I'm only human and respect your opinions.
Please respect mine.

You're not me
you may think differently.
That's ok.

You're not me.
Don't think you're better then me.
Don't try to bring me down.
You don't know what is going on in my life.

You are not me.
But we are the same.

You're not me

I look forward

I look forward.
That is where my future is.
I don't look back where my past is.
I don't need it any more.
I don't stay where I am.
I know I have to look forwards and upwards.

I look forward.
No more staying stuck and wondering *what if*...
I need to go with it and take it slow step by step looking forward.

I look forward.
I take things as they come.
It's time to move on and see life takes me.

I look forward

Letter from the heart

Life is life. It's so true.
We live day in and day out with happy, crazy, sad and even weird moments.
We tell people about our moments.
But we never write a letter from the heart.

Writing a letter from the heart is the most powerful thing ever.
It does not matter what it's about.
It's about you.
But sometimes we forget what we've been through.
We forget till someone reminds us.

Writing a letter from the heart is more powerful than talking to someone.
Now here is where I stop because it will be your letter from your heart not mine.
I'd like you to write why you think it is yours.
There is no wrong answer.
Everyone is different and that makes every letter from the heart so powerful and unique.

Letter from the heart

Can I be who I want to be?

Can I be who I want to be?
Am I just fooling myself?
I've been hiding so long in the shadows
and not used to the light.
Every time I take a step into the light a dark shadow pushes me back.
I know who I am. I want to keep it to myself.
The world is not ready for me.

Can I be who I want to be?
I don't want to be who you want me to be.
Just let me be who I am.
I know why you won't let me be who I am.
I will step out of the dark and into the light where I can be who I am.
I'm in control of myself and will step into that light.

Can I be who I want to be?

The man across the water

walk along a river and suddenly I stop. I look across the water and I see a man looking back at me. The man across the water looks like me, only older. He has the same smile; the same look but so different.

He can see the confusion, happiness and sadness in my face. He has felt it all before. Looking across the water I notice him walking in the same direction as me. I realized that he was walking to his freedom, and me, just half way towards it.

Minutes went by. It felt like hours. I realized my time is precious and need to enjoy it, just like the man across the water who that has done it all before.

Before I started walking again the man spoke to me and said,

"You can do this.
The road may not always be smooth but look at me;
I am the man across the water. I am you."

No more

Time has changed.
Always being the good guy.
Always being taken for granted.
No more.

Too much time wasted on making people happy except for myself.
It's time to take care of myself.
No matter what happens.
You may not think it but I'm important.

It's my time now.
No more thinking.
No more pleasing.
It's time for me.

No more

The wind

The wind is cold and strong.
The wind is an element of power.
The wind can be scary and destructive.
But if wind is a power why don't we see it that way?
The wind can destroy.
The wind is cold.

The wind can be a fresh breeze.
Feel it and accept it as a new beginning.
Let it come over you and take your troubles away, even if it's just for a moment.
The wind can be a positive energy, giving you the extra strength to keep going and not give up.
Feel its power.
Feel its strength.

Most of the time we don't give up on life.
That's the power.
The power of the wind.
The wind being one of the elements might help us to say
"Hey I won't give up".

Listen to the wind.
Even when you can't go on it will say
"Yes you can. I'll blow new energy into you to carry on".
Yes, the wind may not be pretty and nice
but it can also be just what you need.

The wind

Life
Life can be funny sometimes. We go through day by day not really knowing what is in store for us. Not knowing what every new day is going to bring us.

We just walk along a path making choices day by day hoping that they are the right ones. We are never happy. Yes, I can hear a lot of people say, *"I have had happy days"*. I have said the same thing. But how can we be happy if we always complain? We will never be 100% happy.

Yes, sure we laugh, have good and bad moments. We fight; we make up and carry on. We will always do those things. It's natural. It's life. We learn through all our experiences. So yes, life can be funny sometimes. But it's your life so make the best of it.

Let me

Let me be myself as I let you be yourself.
Let me be funny, make jokes, and be made fun of.
Let me make my own mistakes.
Let me fall down and crumble.
I will get up again.
Let me go to my darkest place to find the light again.
Let me but don't stop me.
I don't stop you.

Let me

Can you

Can you tell me how to survive?
Can you feel what I feel?
Can you pick me up when I fall?
Can you really support me?
Can you answer my questions?
I guess you can.

You can tell me how to survive.
You may feel what I feel.
Maybe you can support me and answer all my questions.

Can you feel my soul?
Would you hear it when it cries out for help?
Would you see it?
And would my soul allow it?
Supporting someone when they fall,
answering their questions. It is all so simple to do.

No one can help your soul.
You can't help someone mend a soul.
Your soul will have to mend itself.
The soul is you.

Can you

Untitled

My mind is drifting.
It's going nowhere and everywhere.
So many things are going through my mind.
Nothing settles.
Focusing does not help.
Feeling lost in thoughts with no control over them.
Paralyzed and trapped.
Somewhere I guess.
Nothing I can do but surrender.
And hope my mind will settle.

This shield

I have a shield.
This shield of mine protects me.
But my shield can be broken.
Time and time again I fix it trying to make it strong again.
It holds for a while but then it breaks again.
I keep mending it to make it strong again.

This shield of mine does not give up.
This shield will get stronger every time it breaks.
This shield of mine is my soul.

This shield

Mist

Mist come and goes.
When the mist comes we can't see clearly.
It's too thick.
You can't see what is right in front of you.

It can scare you.
You don't know what is ahead.
You can't see.

You don't know what is on the other side of the mist.
Stay calm.
The mist will go and you will see clearly again.

Mist

Don't want to think any more

Don't want to think any more.
Why can't my head be calm?
I'm telling my mind to give me a break but it won't listen.
It just lets me keep thinking.

At the end of the day I need my mind let me rest.
Sometimes it doesn't.
It all starts again.

Sometimes we need a break from our mind and our thoughts.
Our body gets tired and needs to recharge.
Thinking is painful sometimes.
There is no way out of it but it needs to be done.

Don't want to think any more.

Who am I?

Who am I?
I'm nothing special.
I may be the same as you or maybe not.

I'm not famous.
I may not have the perfect body.
I'm neither rich nor poor.
I struggle everyday as everyone else.
I have my doubts and sometimes feel insecure.

Still trying to find out who I am.
I know what I am supposed to do but I don't act on it.
I'm far behind from where I should be.
That's just me.
Trying to find my way.
I will. Never mind how long it takes.
I will make it to the finish line.
And finally I will know who I really am.

I am letting go

I am letting go.
I can't hold on any longer.
I am letting go.
My hands can't hold the weight any more.

I am letting go.
It does not serve me any longer.
I have tried to hold on for so long but can't do it any more.
The weight is too much.
It's killing me.

It's time to let go and move on.
I am letting go.
I have to.
I will no longer hold on to what I don't need.
And what does not serve me.

I am letting go.

My dear friend

My dear friend, when I first got to know you I kept my distance. When time went by things changed but I still did not let you into my life.

You see my dear friend; I've been there. I trusted someone to be my friend. In the end I was just fooling myself. I was hurt and could not trust or let anybody come close to me again. But, you did.

You, my dear friend, showed me that true friendship still exists. Thanks to you I made more friends. Friends that I never thought I would let in. I still keep my distance sometimes. I still do.

My dear friend, I have many friends now. They care about me and most of all love me for who I am.

My dear friend, thank you for what you have given me. Although my friendship circle has grown there will never be a dear friend like you.

My dear friend

Behind the wall

Behind the wall, we are safe.
Protected from harm and injury
from anything that can hurt us.
It's our safe place to be.

Our wall can be thick and strong.
It can still be damaged.
No matter how many times we are behind the wall the cracks show.
We will always hide behind our wall.
We can rebuild it and show only the things we are comfortable with.
The rest will always be behind the wall.

Wandering

Wandering, roaming around wherever that may be.
Flying, walking, and running towards a destination.
Thoughts and feelings all mixed together
not knowing where it starts or where it ends.

Being in a space having to think and not wanting to.
Wandering, to not be here.
Leaving the real world for as long as it takes.
Wandering, is something we all do.
What can a bit of wandering do for you?

Wandering

Speaking without words

Speak to me.
I listen though you might not hear my answer.
It's not that I'm not giving an answer.
I always do.

I am not here but still close by.
I speak without words.
Let you know I'm there.
I don't need to give you words
or speak with a voice to let you know I'm there.

I speak without words.
Listen and you will hear me.
Listen and you will get my answer.
I am the thought in your head that helps you and guides you.
I speak without words.

Speaking without words

Just let me sleep

Just let me sleep.
I just want to have my eyes closed.
I don't want to see the real world for a minute or so.
Just let me sleep.
I want to keep my eyes closed.
Pretend I'm not here.

I'm fine in the darkness.
I know where the light is.
Let me sleep just for today.
To forget about everything and let sleep will take it away.

Just let me sleep.
I need the rest
to forget about things from the past.
When I wake up my future will be here
And I will have no fear.

Just let me sleep

Hold on

Hold on even if you have nothing left.
When you fight against it all and think there is nothing left,
Look within yourself to find that strength to hold on to.
You will have those moments when you feel like giving up.
That you are defeated, that there is nothing left.

Hold on, you are stronger than you think.
Fight!
Hold on. Don't give up.
You will survive.

Hold on

Love

Love is an amazing feeling.
The first time you meet and you just know.
When the love is pure, you get married
And this will be the most amazing day of your life.
But then everything becomes normal.
Life returns to normal.
I say never lose the passion.
Remember what your partner means to you.
Yes, we go on, and move forward.
But remember your love for that special person
because love never dies.

Love

Story to tell

Everyone is different. Everyone has unique experiences that no one else can claim.

Even when we are in big groups, each person is focusing on something different,
Thinking of something different, noticing something different.

That is why every person has a story to tell, and it is why we can learn from every single person.
We share our stories in the hope that we can help someone.

But as much as we have learned, there is so much that we didn't notice.
Perhaps the person next to us looked up at just the right time to see something we could not.

We listen to other people's stories to discover what we have missed.
Many true stories talk about struggles and difficulties, and can be very sad.
Some true stories can make us laugh as well as cry.
They can be as diverse as any fictional story, and even more powerful because they are true.

Story to tell.

As I lay down and surrender

As I lay down here, I feel like crying. I don't know why.
I have a feeling that I am getting drained. There is no way to stop it.

As I lay down here, I feel like crying. There is nothing I can do.
Trying to keep myself positive saying *"it's just a phase."*

As I lay down here, just fighting what I should not.
Nothing helps but I don't want to give in.

As I lay down here, just surrendering,
Knowing it will be good, knowing it will be painful.

As I lay down here, I surrender to the greater good,
Knowing that my soul needs cleansing.

As I lay down and surrender

Set yourself free

Set yourself free; don't be anyone's prisoner

Set yourself free; don't let anyone hold you back.

Set yourself free; don't let anyone play with your feelings.

You are in control of what happens in your life.
Believe in yourself and leave the rest behind.

Set yourself free; move on.
There are positive things ahead.

Set yourself free.

Dark Clouds

Dark clouds on dark days.
We don't see the light any more
We no longer see the path out of the forest.
The ego gets consumed, thinking about itself.
The beauty in things is not seen any more.
Dark clouds.

Thinking and caring for each other was there.
Hatred has taken over and love has gone.
Is it to late to start over again?
Look at our own mistakes and accept them.
Where is faith? Can we get it back?
Dark clouds.

Darkness has consumed enough.
It's time to let it go.
Return to love. Love is the answer.
Bring back your love into every living thing.
In the end we are all one.
Dark clouds.

Joyful

Close your eyes for a second.
Put a smile on your face.
Be joyful for a life of love and light.

Give a smile to a stranger.
Hug someone everyday
Be joyful for your daily experiences.

Celebrate life and dance with everyone.
Life is too short.
Nobody wants to be alone.

So dream, dare and do.
Share with everybody.
Be joyful.

Life Is Love

From the day we are born we experience love.
From the day your life starts you are loved.
As we grow older love turns into hate
We don't care about each other any more.

Loves gets easily replaced
People don't agree with you, people fight with you.
We all think differently.
Why does it turn into hate?

We can disagree. We can fight. We can argue.
Is it worth breaking up relationships with friends and family?
What about love?
Where is the love we had at the beginning?

Let us not turn love into hate.
And not care about each other any more.
Return to love. Give love.
After all, life is love.

If you knew

If you knew what I was feeling
If you knew what I was thinking
If you knew the secrets of life
Would things be different?
Would you care and do things differently?
Do you listen the moment you feel it inside?

If you knew what pain was all about.
If you knew things would be different
If you knew you could bare it
Would you recognize it?
Would you keep the secrets to yourself?
Do you share it?

If you knew would you change anything?

Memories

Can you remember?
Do you want to remember?
We can't remember everything.
We are only human.

We remember what happened not so long ago.
We remember good things.
But we don't remember everything.
Our memory fails sometimes.
We forget what happened.
Or do we just want to forget?

We won't always remember our memories.
That's ok.
It's more important that they happened
and left a mark in our life.

No matter how big or small
No matter how bad or good.

They are yours.

Memories.

Hurt me

Hurt me.
I can take the pain.
Hurt me.
I can handle it.

I will carry it.
My back is big enough.
I will feel the sorrow.
I will feel the pain.

Hurt me.
I will cry alone.
Hurt me. Break me.
I will get up.

My pain hurts but it won't last.
I am strong.
Stronger than the hurt you've given me.

Hurt me.
I will get over it.
Your hurt will make me stronger.

Hurt me

You're my secret

You're my secret.
You live deep inside.
When you rise to the surface, I forget who I am.
I break all the rules.
Rules I put in place for myself.

I tell myself I can't do this anymore.
I want to change so badly.
But you, my little secret, flare up again.
Knowing you can change things only for a few minutes.

Yes, you get the job done.
Taking me to that dark place again.
A place I don't want to be.
But your words almost control me.
You're my secret.
One day I will break you, my little secret.

You're my secret

I've had enough

I've had enough.
I won't take it any more.
I have given you control for too long.
Today I am taking my life back.

For many years you've taken control.
Not any more.
I was strong then. I am strong now.
You don't have power over me.
I am not a puppet doing what you want.

I have a choice.
I have to be respected.
I have a mind.
Don't control me
I won't let you any longer.
I've had enough and will stand up for what I believe.

I've had enough.

Set yourself free

It stops right here. Right now.
It's time to set yourself free.
You have been played with long enough.
It's time not to take it any longer.

Today is the day you take your life back.
Do what you want.
It's time to set yourself free.
No more pressure.
No more the obligations.

It stops here. Right now.
Time to set yourself free.
Don't care what others think.
Decide what you want to do.
Nobody deserves to be controlled.
It stops today.

Set yourself free.

Today

Today I fell down.
Today I had enough.
Today I broke down.
Today I was too tired to fight.
Today I gave up.

Tomorrow I will be back.
I will be strong again.
I will fight whatever comes my way.

Today let me be weak.
Today let me make sense of what is happening.
Let me have today.
Let me stand on the sidelines of my life.
Let me see what I no longer need.
I just need today.

Today

I am here

I am here.
What happens from this *here moment* is up to me.
Do I want to stay were I am?
Do I move on?
Should I stay in my comfort zone?
Should I explore further?
Am I happy in my *here moment*?
Do I choose just to stay here for a while and then move on?
I am here.
I have time to decide what my next step will be.
What will you do in your *here moment*?

I am here

Words from beyond

We are always here.
It may not be here physically but we are with you.
We have not forgotten you and never will.
We still care about you and are here for you in times of need.
You just don't see the signs.
We let you know that we are near you.
You brush it off thinking you've imagined it.
We send you signs that leave you wondering.
We are near you.

Words from beyond.

We connect with you through dreams.
That's how we really connect.
Know you are never alone.
We are right beside you.
Meditate and connect with us.
Enjoy life and learn.
Know we always love you.
We are not here physically but we have not disappeared.
We are near you.

Words from beyond.

Lights out

Every night the lights go out.
We go to sleep.
We know another day will be waiting.
We face another day.
Another day full of hope,
new beginnings and second chances.

Sometimes we succeed.
Sometimes we fail.
When we fail, our lights go out.
We support people who have failed;
we talk with them,
struggle with them
fight with them
Hoping they see the light again.

The message is clear; help where you can.
Pull back when it gets too much.
Never give up.
Everyone deserves to live in the light

Lights out

I think back

I think back at the moments we shared.
I think back because that's all I have left.
How did we become strangers?
After all these years our friendship is gone.

You're not in my life any longer
But sometimes I think back.
Back to what we did.
We can't turn back time.
We need to move on.
It's ok to think back.
Think back but don't dwell on the past.
Think forward about new things to come.

I think back

One request

One request is all I ask.
One request that should not be ignored.
One request, difficult yet simple.
One request, you're not even trying.

You carry out request for others.
Why not mine?
One request, it's a battle every day.
It shouldn't be.
Is one request so hard?
One request, but nothing happens.
What does it take to get you to make one request happen?

All I ask is

One request

Copyright © 2018 Paul Kuypers. All rights reserved.

Game over

You convinced me and I fell for it.
You convinced me and I played the game.

Everything has changed.
Cruel is what you did.
Cruel is what you're doing.

But today everything changes.
Today it's game over.

Today is the day I take control.
It's game over.

Your game ends here and now.
You've had me under your control for too long.
It's over.
I am not your toy any more.

This game you lose.

Game over.